HOW TO HEAL WITH CRYSTALS AND CRYSTAL GRIDS

BY EL KA

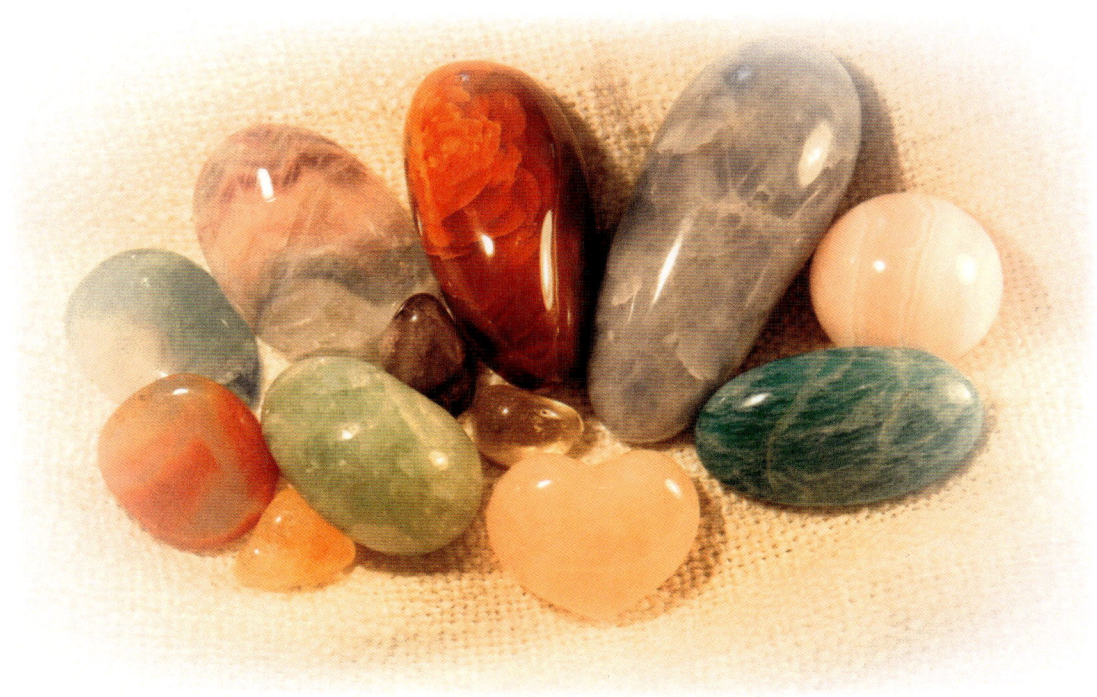

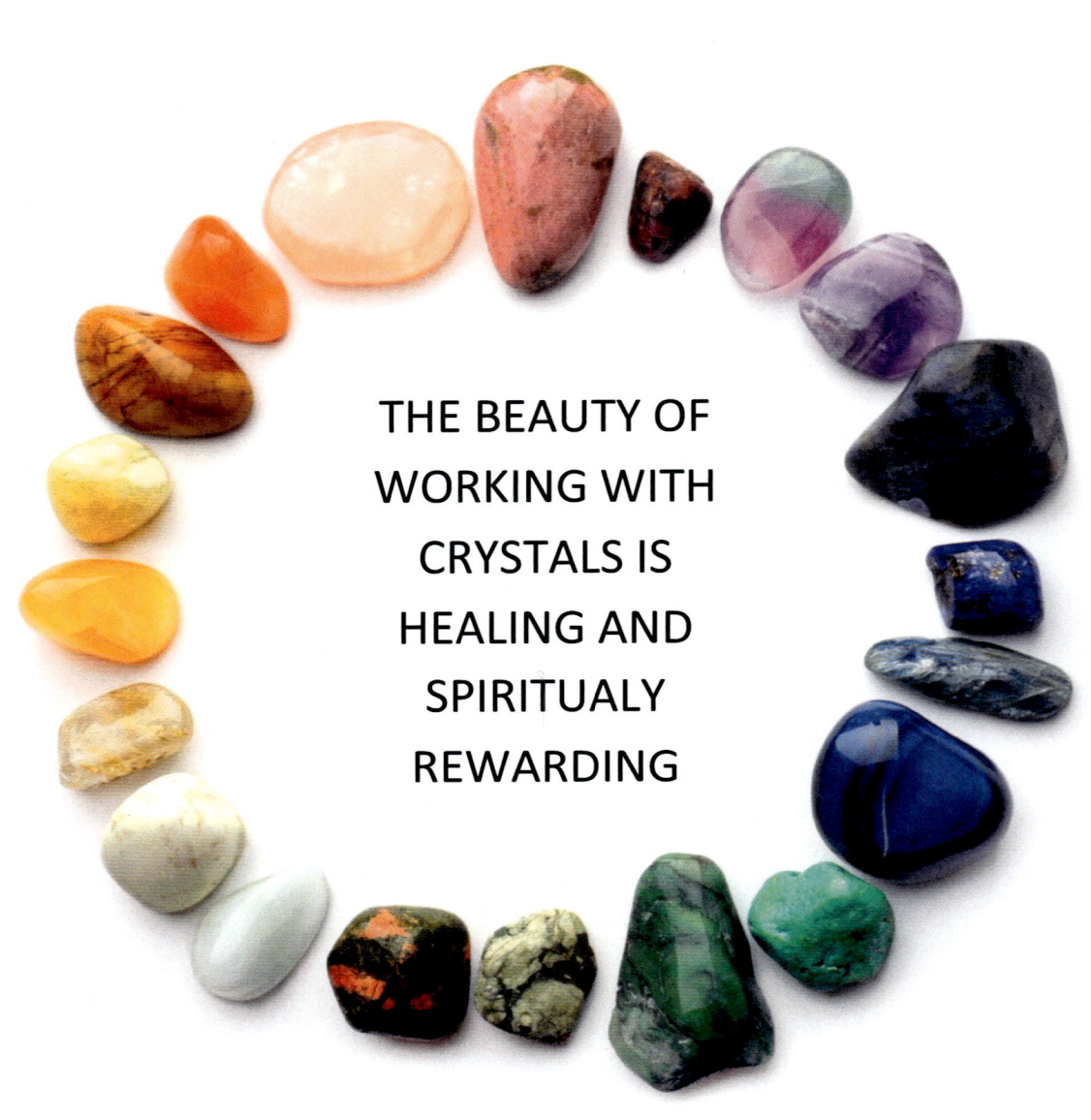

THE BEAUTY OF WORKING WITH CRYSTALS IS HEALING AND SPIRITUALY REWARDING

EL KA © 2014 - 2021

All rights reserved. No part of this publication may be reproduced or transmitted in any form or by any means, electronic, mechanical, photocopying, recording or otherwise.

DISCLAIMER:
The information in this book does not constitute any medical advice, nor is it intended to take the place of medical or psychological treatment. It is not intended to act as a replacement of any legal or other expert advice. Every effort and attempt to ensure that this book includes accurate information has been made on the part of the author, however mistakes and / or inaccuracies may well exist. The author accepts no liability or responsibility for any loss or damage caused or thought to be caused by the advice or information provided in this book. It is recommended that any advice given in this book be used in conjunction with other medical and expert advice.

http://elenaka.wix.com/crystalgridcreations

BY EL KA

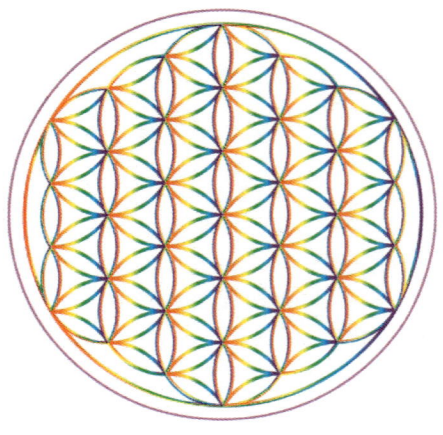

HOW TO HEAL WITH CRYSTALS AND CRYSTAL GRIDS

TABLE OF CONTENTS | HOW TO HEAL WITH CRYSTALS AND CRYSTAL GRIDS

Foreword   9

Part One: What are Crystals and How They Work

Introduction	13
What are Crystals? How do they Work?	15
History of Crystals?	15
What are the Benefits of Crystals?	16
Healing People with Crystals?	17
Choosing & Buying Crystals?	19
How to Cleanse Crystals?	23
Handling Crystals	26
How to Activate and Program Your Crystals?	26
Meditating with Crystals?	27
How Crystals Correspond to Earth Elements?	38

Part Two: Crystal Grids and How They Work

What is a Crystal Grid? How do they Work?	44
What are the Benefits of Crystal Grids?	44
Power of Your Mind with Conjunction of Crystal Grids	45
Manifesting Goals Technique	46
Birthstones & Zodiac Gemstone Associations	56
Types of Crystals to use for Grids?	58
Sacred Geometry & Types of Bases to use for Grids?	58
Instructions for Creating Crystal Grids?	59
Here Are a Few Tips about Crystal Grids	61
Other Layouts for Crystal Grids	62
What are Body Crystal Grids? How do they Work?	63
Seal of Solomon/Star of David Grid	65
Amethyst Healing Layout	67
Aches & Pains Layout	68
Easing PMT & Menstrual Cramps	69
Amethysts for Headaches	70
Foot Layout	71
Chakra Layout	72
Explanation of the Chakra Purposes	74
Crystals & Essential Oils for Chakra Balancing	75
Empowering Affirmations to use for Chakra Clearing	82
Practical Grid Recipes & Formations	83

Part Three: Healing Wands, What They are and How They Work

What are Wands? How are they Made?	137
Healing Methods with Crystal Wands?	137
How to Choose a Wand?	138

TABLE OF CONTENTS | HOW TO HEAL WITH CRYSTALS AND CRYSTAL GRIDS

Process of Getting to Know Your Wand?	139
How to Program a Crystal Wand?	139
How to Cleanse and Recharge a Crystal Wand?	140
How to Heal with a Wand?	140
Sweeping Away Built Up Energies From the Auric Field?	142
Pictures of Various Healing Wands	143

Part Four: What are Gemstone Elixirs and How to Make Them

How to Make Gemstone Elixirs	154
Preserving the Gemstone Elixir	156
Dosage of How much to Take of a Gem Elixir	156
How to Use Gemstone Elixirs	156
Empower Your Gemstone Elixir	157
Gemstone Elixir Recipes	157
Charging Crystals after Gemstone Elixir	158
Potentially Toxic or Harmful Crystals	158
Safety Guidelines for Using Crystals for Making Gem Elixirs	162

Part Five: Working with Pendulums to Heal Chakras

Working with Pendulums to Heal the Chakras	167
Choosing a Pendulum	167
Cleansing a Pendulum	167
Recharging a Pendulum	168
Getting to Know a Pendulum	168
Preparing for a Healing	168
Holding the Pendulum	168
Going over the Chakras	168
Allowing the Pendulum to Move	169
Explanation of the Pendulum Movements	170
Healing a Blocked Chakra Point	170
Cleansing the Pendulum & the Healer When Finished	170

Index

Crystal Properties & Uses	175

Appendix I

Crystal Healing Grid Nets	345

Appendix II

Assembling Crystals for a Healing Kit	350
How to Transport Crystals	351
References	353

FOREWARD

This book seeks to explore the ways in how to work with crystals for various healing modalities. To expand the boundaries of the mind and imagination in order to discover the health benefits of using crystals, from the past way of healing to present day techniques.

In *How to Heal with Crystals and Crystal Grids*, EL KA has delved into one of the gaps in the field of crystal healing to change the concept of some confusion regarding using crystals for healing modalities and seeks to educate, illuminate, and bring clarity to crystal grids as well as other crystal healing techniques. Throughout the book there is information provided on what crystals are and how to work with crystals in healing the body with crystal pendulums, wands, crystal grids, and manifestation techniques for achieving your goals along with life accomplishments. The book will teach you about how to heal and cleanse the chakras, meditation, create physical crystal body grids, and explore all you want to know about crystals.

Whether you are new to crystals or an experienced practitioner you will find something new here to inform and stimulate the mind.

Perhaps it is the way EL KA presents the research methods behind crystal grids and other forms of crystal healing, along with keeping this information approachable to the enthusiast as well as the expert reader that adds a sense of a well-rounded method of education to this book.

EL's step by step guide to crystal healing and practical detailed information about this topic are the fundamentals for why this book is easy to understand and a joy to follow.

This is the type of book that offers the reader an idea to explore the possibilities of life, creates a thought and gives hope for positive outcomes. The book also points you on the directed path so you can travel the same enlightened road to whichever destination you are destined to reach.

Whether you need prosperity, protection, or want to bring healing to people, animals, or Mother Nature within the following pages of this book you will find ideas to stimulate your mind and healing methods to follow.

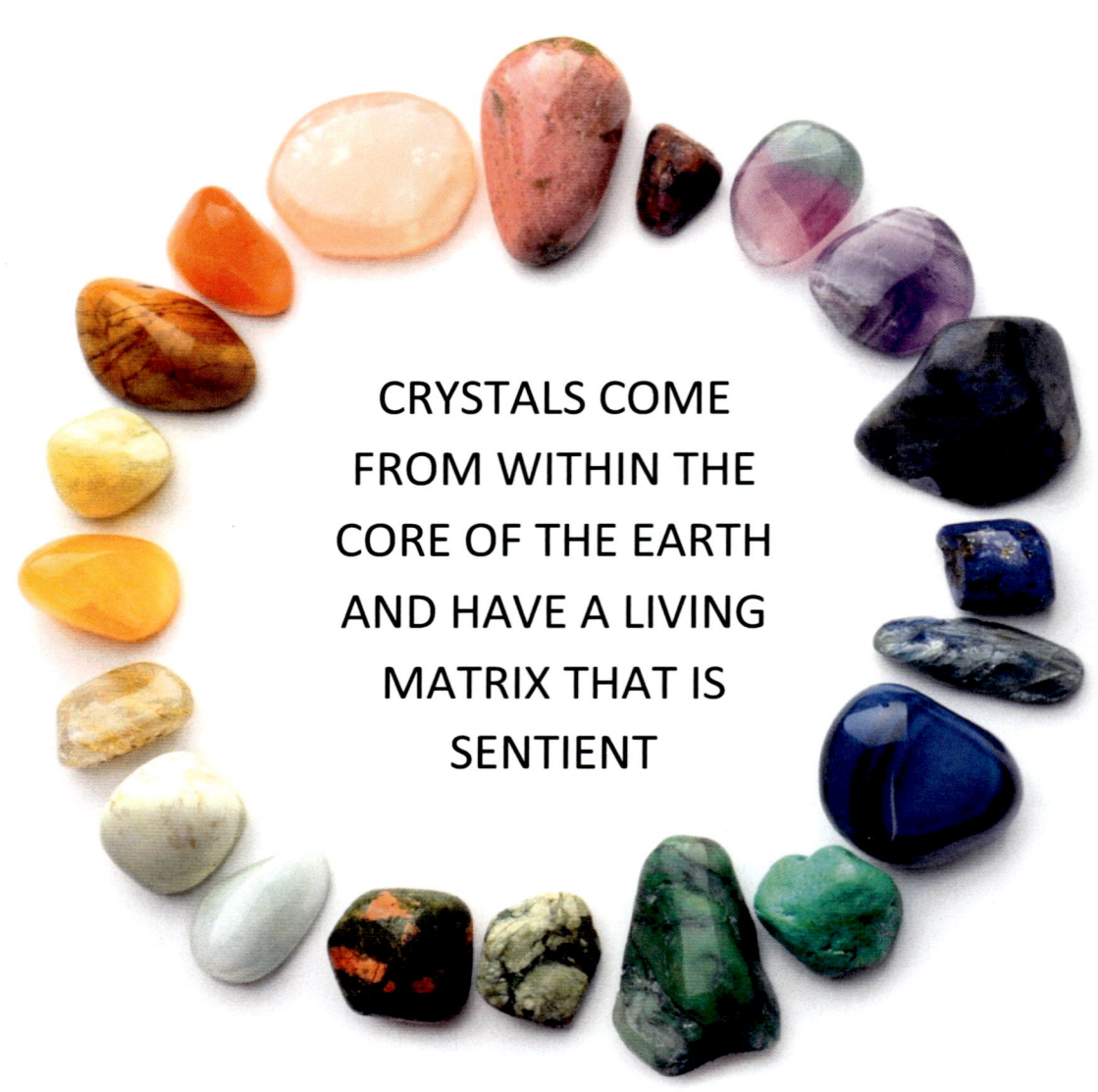

CRYSTALS COME FROM WITHIN THE CORE OF THE EARTH AND HAVE A LIVING MATRIX THAT IS SENTIENT

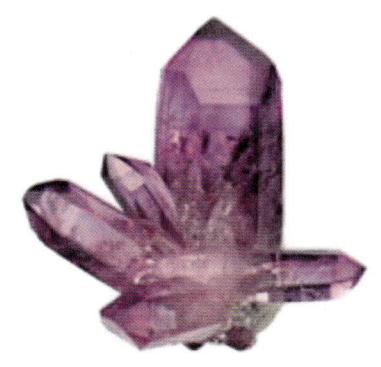

PART ONE

WHAT ARE CRYSTALS AND HOW THEY WORK

INTRODUCTION

I have been interested in crystals for a while now since I was a young woman going up to the mountains and selecting beautiful specimens while walking in the forest, up the mountain slopes, beaches, and visiting crystal shops on my journeys.

During high school I took an Earth science class and discovered that crystals come from the Earth growing in interesting formations and having different properties from which they are made. That was the scientific explanation behind crystals that I knew. I enjoyed the beauty of the crystals and stones that I collected but had no idea that there was so much more to these living creations.

As I got older, I started discovering the healing benefits of crystals. I learned that crystals and stones have the abilities to help improve a person's health, manifest goals, etc. through the creation of crystal grids where the crystals are put on the grids and the person works with them. This technique has helped me to greatly improve my own health both physically, and psychologically, therefor making me a lot happier in my life. My spiritual path of enlightenment has also been revealed to me by choosing to work with crystals. I have become much more grounded and comfortable with who I am as a person, being secure in my role as a crystal healer on Earth.

I have also worked with making body grids where I put crystals around a client's body and let the crystals heal the client. When I work with the body grids I use wands in conjunction to the crystals in order to balance out the client's chakras and auric field.

For this book I decided to write about the history of crystals, what they are, how to use crystal grids, meditating with crystals, work with body grids, wands, gem elixirs, and also pendulums. All of these are healing modalities that involve working with crystals on a deeply profound level.

I have a lot of knowledge about healing with different alternative medicine modalities and working on being spiritually balanced and I wanted to share these experiences in this book.

My educational background includes being a Reiki Master, Crystal Healer, Shamanic Practitioner, and an Intuitive. In all these modalities there is the aspect of working with crystals, and spirituality. I drew on this knowledge to help write this book.

By my personality trait, I am a self-learner who has worked in a university library finding facts along with valuable knowledge. I like researching the various healing medicinal modalities having to do with crystals, so I gathered the facts for this book from my experiences and other research sources which greatly contributed to providing information for this project.

I hope readers enjoy learning about crystals and the different alternative medicine modalities that incorporate healing with the use of crystals.

Facts about Crystals:

What are Crystals? How do they Work?

Crystals are precious or semi-precious gemstone minerals that grow from the earth. Crystal formations contain the most orderly and stable structures in the natural world. The atoms and molecules in crystals form regular repeating patterns called a crystalline lattice. These structured lattices form symmetrical repeating arrays which create the foundation of the crystals. The vibrational energetic properties of crystals and their highly stable structures are ideal for healing purposes and for crystal grids.

The perfect order of the crystal lattices is created due to the individual atoms and molecules being packed together as tightly as possible during crystal growth; this is partly because of strong electro-magnetic forces and high pressures around the crystals as they form. This stability ensures that crystals react in characteristic, precise and predictable ways to a broad spectrum of energies, including sound, light, heat and pressure - this is why they are of use in the electronics industry.

As researched by firsthand experience from the author of this book, crystals can respond to bioelectricity and consciousness (i.e. to thought and emotion) and there is evidence that they have a consciousness of their own. Crystals are highly evolved within the Mineral world and are directed to work with humanity for the higher good and for the growth advancement of all the Kingdoms on Earth. By applying the stable and focused energy of crystals to dysfunctional energy systems within the human body, a state of balance and optimum health can be restored. Since crystals have high vibrational energies, they can raise and uplift the auric fields of humanity to help with speeding up the healing process in the body and also help to cure ailments.

The healing properties of crystals cannot be easily diminished as the crystals have strong reservoirs of energy that is being drawn from the universe, this pure light energy is regularly replenished when the crystals are cleansed as needed. Quartz crystals resonate with the liquid crystals that are found to be within the physical body, and can transfer their energies to the bloodstream for health and rejuvenation, as well as transmuting unwanted information that may be locked within bodily tissues or the mind and other etheric bodies. When crystals are used in geometrical arrays they have an amplified effect, which can be put to different uses depending on the nature of the stones chosen and their placements.

An interesting fact to know is that crystals can retain and re-transmit our thoughts as some of them are record keepers. This phenomenon is similar to the technology of magnetic storage on a computer.

History of Crystals?

Crystals have been used for healing for thousands of years. Research has shown that crystals go as far back as to the lost city of Atlantis which Edgar Cayce a famous psychic healer showcased in his books and written papers. In the Far Eastern and Native American cultures crystals have been used for not only helping in physical healing but also in spiritual rituals. The crystals are used in modern healings by shamans and crystal healers to realign the energies of a person's auric field through doing a chakra cleanse, or a crystal grid on or around the human body. During healings crystals are also intuitively programmed to help people to deal with emotional blockages that can be resonating from the soul and the brain. The crystals work on purifying and removing these emotional blockages as well as clearing away energetic trauma that can cause physical ailments.

The first known reference to the healing power of crystals comes from an Egyptian papyrus dated around 1600 BC which gives directions for their use. This information comes from the Ultimate Crystal Healing Guide book by Louis Waweru.

In ancient times beads of lapis lazuli, malachite, and red jasper were worn around a sick person's neck so that the disease could pass through the beads and disappear. This method of healing is still practiced today, where people wear pendants, earrings, rings, and bracelets made from crystals to heal the emotional state and the physical body. The practice of placing or wearing stones on various areas of the body was only part of the repertoire of healers in history. A popular medicinal method that had been utilized was to pulverize gems, then mix the gem powder with a liquid, and drink it. This is similar to the crystal remedies which are used today called gem elixirs, but the crystals are left in the filtered or mineral water so that their energy pattern can be imprinted on the water, the crystal is then removed and then the 'charged' water is bottled for drinking. This method cannot be done with all crystals though, as some are highly toxic, like for example pyrite, hematite, malachite, etc. Some common types of crystals that can be used in gem elixirs are amethyst, rose quartz, citrine, clear quartz, and aventurine. Consult a gem elixirs recipe book to see which crystals are toxic and which are not, it is a good idea to consult more than one source to verify this information.

It has been historically documented that crystals have been used to make different types of either stone grids like Stonehenge or some are largely built sacred geometry structures like the Great Pyramid at Giza placed strategically on the ground with the possible purpose of connecting with the ley-lines of the Earth. These ley-lines are the planetary equivalent of the meridian channels in people and are a web of energetic grid lines creating a type of power matrix that allows some people to tune into light-information stimulating the higher consciousness within themselves which connects with advanced knowledge from the universal grid of life. All these stone grids are centers of spiritual energy for healing of humanity and the Earth.

An interesting fact to know is that our earth is 85% crystal. The earth's crust is largely made from silicon and oxygen, combined with six other elements, aluminum, iron, calcium, sodium, potassium and magnesium. Scientists have discovered that from this combination comes the awe inspiring variety of crystal colors, shapes, sizes and hardness.

What are the Benefits of Crystals?

1. Crystals help to relieve headaches, ailments, physical aches, and pains on the body.
2. Healing energy from crystals helps to restore the human cells and organs to optimum functioning levels, like blood disorders, stomach issues, and throat issues.
3. The healing properties of crystals help to restore health to people, animals, and Mother Nature. Crystals can be placed on people and animals to relieve pain, as well the crystals can be put out in the garden or out in nature where healing is needed for the earth. This can be in a form of a crystal grid or just having crystals surrounding the space. A crystal grid can also be made to represent a person or animal as a holographic projection to provide them with healing.

4. Crystals help to remove energetic blockages from the human body so a person is at their optimum health, this can be done through various crystal healing techniques like a chakra cleanse, body crystal grids, crystal body massage, or crystal meditation.
5. Crystals help with mood improvement, to change negative thought patterns of the brain into positive ways of thinking in order to improve people's lives in achieving happiness and having healthier lifestyles.
6. Crystals have protective properties that help to remove negative energies from environments like homes, businesses, etc., and to cleanse the spaces so the bad energies do not return.
7. Crystals can help with intuitive work, like psychic development, finding inner wisdom, or having a gut feeling hunch to sometimes ask the crystals questions and then get answers for hard to solve situations. Many types of crystals bring in the healing process in order to create peace, calmness, and stability into people's lives. Crystals can also help with manifesting spiritual awakening and gifts in metaphysical abilities like the ability to create fire without matches, call in water, or air when needed, etc.

Healing People with Crystals?

From healing research done on people it has been shown that crystals relate to body parts just as energetic chakras, muscles and teeth do.

For example, if someone has a problem with a tooth, be it toothache, or a tooth infection, or even when someone just chips a tiny piece off from a tooth while eating something hard, a person will likely have pain in their mouth. A small tumbled fluorite crystal can help relieve the pain. Fluorite helps to strengthen bone tissue, especially the teeth; it eases bone tissue pain, and helps to alleviate dental diseases. The tumbled fluorite crystal may be put into the mouth between the jaw and the sore tooth. After a couple of minutes remove the fluorite from your mouth. Cleanse the fluorite with healing though energy and wash it under clean cold water. Put it back into your mouth again. Do this a total of three times. This method of easing the pain from a sore tooth, also works with using hematite.

Another example of where crystals can be used is to relieve headaches. The first step is to find out what is causing the headache. There are many different types of headaches. What type of headache is it, a migraine, or is it stress related, or is it food/drink related? If the headache is stress related then amethyst or amber can be placed on the brow or forehead area and they will relieve the pain. However, if the pain is food/drink related, a crystal which calms the stomach will be needed. Such crystals are amethyst, carnelian, green fluorite, garnet and jet.

At times headaches and other diseases can be caused not by our own bodies but by outside influences which are connected to environmental factors such as geopathic stress and electromagnetic smog which can come from sources like wireless internet connection, electrical lighting, recording devices, etc. If this happens then your home can be cleared of these energies by having a Himalayan salt lamp placed at your desk, or beside your TV to cancel out these negative energies. It is a good idea to turn off electromagnetic sources at night so they do not emit negative energies into your environment. As well where there are good points of energy in homes, it is recommended to place an amethyst nearby to radiate the positive energy out to the rest of the house. On occasion more than one type of crystal may be needed at the same time to amplify positive energy. In these instances, care should be taken in what crystals are used in conjunction with each other. An important fact to keep in mind is that some crystals support and complement each other but they can also cancel each other out. Amethyst and rose quartz complement each other in removing negative energies from spaces. Citrine and carnelian also complement each other in relieving stress and anxiety.

Here is a Chart of Healing Crystals:

AGATE – A variety of Chalcedony. Calming; comforting and useful for relieving pain.	**AMAZONITE** – A variety of Felspar. Aphrodisiac; soothes nervous system and strengthens the heart.	**AMBER** – Fossilized pine tree resin. Electrifying; relieves fear, depression, tiredness, asthma & infections.
AMETHYST – A variety of Quartz. Protects against excesses in all forms. Calming; powerful blood cleanser; excellent for meditation.	**AQUA AURA** – Calms the emotional body and heals holes in the auric field. Activates and cleanses the chakras. Helps to attract wealth and success and good for aiding with spiritual growth.	**AQUAMARINE** – A variety of Beryl. Keeps one young and happy; calms nerves; helps banish fear and phobias; excellent for meditation; good luck for travelers.
AVENTURINE – A variety of Quartz. Improves creativity, perception and independence; alleviates anxiety; helps relieve fears; encourages a positive attitude.	**AZURITE** – A Copper Carbonate. Increases sensitivity, amplifies natural healing abilities; strengthens blood; helps body utilize oxygen. Effective in bone diseases, arthritis, etc.	**BLOODSTONE** – A variety of Quartz. Used to balance and calm the uneasy mind; helps to develop courage and caution; augments mental and physical vitality; powerful physical healer.
CALCITE – A Calcium Carbonate. Alleviates fear and reduces stress; valued as a thought amplifier; increases capacity for astral projection; aids kidneys; pancreas and spleen.	**CARNELIAN** – A variety of Chalcedony. Energizes blood; aids kidneys, lungs, gallbladder and pancreas; increases faith and repels fear; helps alleviate bad temper and brings contentment.	**CHRYSOCOLLA** – Gem Silica. Strengthens lungs and thyroid gland; enhances metabolism. Is helpful for nervous tension, fear, guilt, ulcers and digestive imbalance. Excellent for female disorders; activates feminine qualities.
CHRYSOPRASE – A variety of Quartz. Eases depression; helpful for sexual imbalance and fertility; maybe helpful in stabilizing blood pressure and relieves bleeding.	**CITRINE** – A variety of Quartz. Relieves tiredness; brings happiness; strengthens nerves; good for heart, kidneys and liver. Enhances body healing energy and tissue regeneration.	**COPPER** – Influences blood flow; aids metabolism; balances emotions; alleviates poor memory and the ability to retain thoughts; eases arthritic pain.
DIAMOND – A master healer. Enhances brain function; draws toxicity from the body; useful for anxiety, insecurity and low self-esteem; thought amplifier.	**EMERALD** – A variety of Beryl. Calms the troubled mind; increases psychic clairvoyance; helps mental alertness.	**FLOURITE** – Calcium Fluoride. Strengthens bone tissue, especially teeth; eases bone tissue and dental diseases; alleviates anxiety and sexual frustration.
GARNET – Enhances the willpower and perseverance; comforts when depressed; eases bad dreams.	**GOLD** – Balances brain hemispheres; aids tissue regeneration; eases depression; amplifies thoughts and aids thought retention.	**HEMATITE** – Iron Oxide. Increases resistance to stress; alleviates low self-esteem; balances male/female qualities; good for all blood disorders.
HERKIMER DIAMOND – A variety of Quartz. Powerful amplifier; releases stress and tension; relaxes muscles; increases awareness of dreams.	**JASPER** – A variety of Chalcedony. Helps morning sickness; helpful for dealing with stomach, liver and kidney problems; calms uneasy minds.	**KUNZITE** – A variety of Spodumene. Very high lithium content which is helpful in cases of depression and mental disorders; aids in longevity; emotional balancer; has soothing and calming qualities.
KYANITE – Promotes good communication and helps to create loyalty, and fair treatment to others. Aligns the chakras and subtle bodies, clearing pathways and meridians on the body.	**LAPIS LAZULI** – A variety of Sodium. Releases tension and anxiety; helpful for dealing with throat and eye problems. This is a friendship stone which strengthens love and gives self-confidence.	**MAGNETITE** – Iron Oxide. Helps in cases of dizziness, headaches and insomnia; used in dentistry manifestation. Good for dealing with sports injuries, bruises, sprains, muscle and joint pain and stiffness.
MALACHITE – a Copper Carbonate. Used to promote sleep; helpful in cases of arthritis, rheumatism and menstrual disorders; useful for neurological disorders and visual problems.	**MOONSTONE** – A variety of Felspar. Brings success and contentment; protects against accidents; benefits pregnancy & menstrual disorders and stimulates lactation.	**OBSIDIAN** – A volcanic glass. Balances the stomach, intestines and muscle tissue. Helps alleviate inflammation and reduces stress. Protects soft-hearted and gentle people.
OPAL – The friendship stone. Emotional balancer used for radiating sex appeal; amplifies thought; eases sexual depression.	**PERIDOT** – Olivine. Strengthens the heart and eyes; aids tissue regeneration.	**PYRITE** – Iron Sulphide. Alleviates nervous exhaustion and stammering; eases anxiety; aids the digestion; enhances brain function.
QUARTZ CRYSTAL – Clear. Conquers fear; protects against loss of balance, and motion sickness; balances emotions and stimulates the brain function; excellent for meditation.	**RHODOCHROSITE** – A variety of Manganese. Enhances intellectual powers; strengthens self-identity and lessens nightmares; helps to heal emotional wounds.	**ROSE QUARTZ** – The Love Stone. Aids creative thinking; stimulates artistic ability; eases sexual and emotional unbalances; reduces stress; enhances forgiveness and relaxation.
RUTILATED QUARTZ – Stimulates damaged parts of the brain; strengthens the immune system; increases clairvoyance; eases depression.	**SAPPHIRE** – Transparent blue gemstone. A variety of Corundum. Stimulates telepathy, astral projection, clairvoyance; strengthens the heart and kidneys; stimulates the desire for prayer and inner peace.	**SELENITE** – A variety of Gypsum. Strengthens the bones and teeth; rejuvenates the prostate gland, testicles and uterus; helps to release tension; activates higher creativity.
SERPENTINE – A variety of Magnesium. Balances female qualities; alleviates paranoia; increases psychic abilities; stimulates the heart, kidneys, lungs, pituitary and the thymus glands.	**SMOKY QUARTZ** – Increases fertility; assists with heart problems; muscular deterioration; aids depression; good for meditation.	**SODALITE** – A variety of Sodium. Relieves subconscious fears & guilt; stimulates metabolism; balances the thyroid; enhances communication and creative expression.
TIGER EYE – A variety of Chalcedony. Assists with having healthier thoughts, aids in mental faculties and literacy; balances emotions and stubbornness.	**TOPAZ** – An Aluminum Silicate. Balances the emotions, improves the appetite and sense of taste; strengthens the thyroid gland; detoxifies the body; helps with relaxing and bringing in a state of calmness.	**TOURMALINE** – A variety of Boro-silicate. Builds self-confidence and concentration; good for nervousness and sadness; gives inspiration; aids sleep; vitalizes the energetic fields; good for infections. Good for lowering cholesterol and high blood pressure.

Refer to the above chart of healing crystals to figure out how the healing properties of the crystals correlate with helping to heal emotional and physical symptoms of ailments. These crystals are meant to help with activating the natural healing processes of the body but they in no way replace the traditional medical system and medication. They can be used in conjunction with traditional medicine to help with speeding up the healing process where needed.

How to Select and Utilize Certain Crystals?

Choosing & Buying Crystals?

Crystal healer practitioners can select the crystals they need purely using logic, by choosing specific stones for a specific purpose or condition as shown in a crystal directory or book. However the healers need to bear in mind that how a crystal's energies interact with each of them will often vary subtly.

Alternatively healers may select their crystals using their own intuition, by working through instinct and inner guidance or by "gut feeling". This means choosing a crystal, taking it into their hands and holding the crystal they are drawn to; the first one the healer really notices or that they want to pick up. If selecting a crystal for a specific ailment or purpose, or to give to another person, the healer needs to know about that ailment, keeping the purpose or person in mind when starting their selection process, and focus on it throughout. It is important to keep in mind that each person may feel and get different things from the same crystal, for the vibrational interaction of each person's energy field with a crystal's energetic frequency is always unique.

As an optional method, the crystal healer can choose their crystals through mechanics, by backing up their "gut feelings" with a tangible test such as dowsing or muscle testing (kinesiology). When using a dowser (crystal pendulum) or muscle testing the healer needs to be grounded, centered, clear and focused for the results to be accurate and reliable, but this can provide supportive input to a person's intuitive thoughts and feelings, therefore it can be a useful option until the healer has the confidence to trust fully in their intuition.

Take notice of the sensations you get when handling the crystal. Does the energy vibration of the crystal resonate positively with your own body energy field? It is important to feel connected with the crystal you are holding, and feel contentment, peace, and happiness when working with the crystal. If the crystal does not resonate with you and has a heavy energy field to it then perhaps consider choosing another crystal that works better with your energies.

During the selection process of finding crystals keep in mind about the types of finishes you would like the crystals to have whether you want cut or uncut crystals, polished or rough stones. Consider the shape and size of the crystals; whether it is comfortable to hold them in a person's hand in order to easily work with the selected crystals. How heavy or large are the crystals, and how long time wise can a person hold them in their hands. For healers to do precise work with crystals, the crystals selected need to have clarity, purity, and a degree of perfection not having damage like cracks, fractures, or breaks to faces and points on the crystals.

When purchasing crystals be careful of buying fake crystals especially clear quartz spheres, sometimes sellers may offer glass instead of the real quartz on the internet. Buy your crystals from reputable sources like physical crystal stores and ask questions about the crystals you are purchasing so you know where they came from. If buying crystals online you obviously cannot hold them before buying them, or exactly feel how their energy vibrates with yours. That does not mean you cannot buy crystals online. Take a moment quietly and ask your higher self or your intuition "Is this the right crystal for me at this time, do I really need it". If the answer you sense is yes, it feels right, then go ahead and buy the crystal(s). On the other hand if you feel negativity about the crystal then pass over it, and look for another crystal to buy until you get positive feedback. It is important to look at the product images to make sure the crystals do not have any obvious mayor flaws or damage, if the pictures of the crystals are clearly easy to view then they will show if the crystals are nice looking or if there are cracks, dents, breaks, etc. Have a look at the product description and see if the crystal is new, used, etc. Check the seller ratings, if there is too much negative feedback about products then maybe look for better sellers to buy from. Look at the information from which country the crystals are being shipped from, and reviews on how reliable the shipping is from other customers, if too many reviews say that items never arrived, it is a good idea to buy something else similar to what you were looking for from more reputable sellers. Sometimes the crystals look very beautiful in the online photos, and in person are nothing as described in the online images, for example the item is damaged, color is wrong, the shape or size of item is way off the scale, or it is something completely different from what was originally being offered in the deal. If this happens and the item that arrived is not as described insist and ask for a refund of your full money back as most online sales from places like Ebay, or Etsy have buyer protection if using PayPal to pay for crystal specimens. This can make a big difference when buying quality crystals and can save time and money when making buying choices.

There are many different types of crystals to choose from when making purchase selections. Some examples are small tumble stones, palm stones, crystal eggs, clusters, hearts, merkabas, skulls, spheres, pyramids, obelisks, wands, points, geodes, etc. The shapes, forms, and sizes of crystals are endless in abundance as there are hundreds of crystals in existence and a lot of lapidary stores which sell them.

From personal experience of buying crystals there are special kinds of crystals that have inclusions, rainbows, unusual formations, and special features. In the below diagrams are a few examples of these types of crystals.

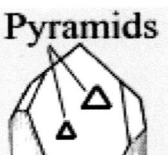

Record Keepers

The special features of unique crystals include being a record keeper crystal which is excellent at absorbing and retaining information so it is a memory keeper. Often times record keeper crystals already have stored information that is meant to be accessed by the owner who buys the crystal and they deal with a specific lesson that a person needs to learn. Record keeper crystals usually appear in clear quartz, smoky quartz, or amethyst and they have one or more raised triangles that are located on the face of the crystal, these triangles look like pyramids.

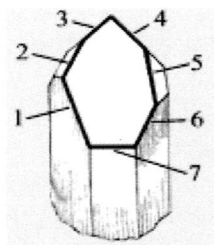

Channeling Crystals

There are also channeling crystals that have seven edges surrounding the largest sloping face of the crystal. Channeling crystals are usually clear quartz; they are useful for obtaining information deep from within a person's psyche or from sources that are outside of a person's normal realm. The channeling crystals can help people to draw on the knowledge and information that is provided by the universe, and can aid people in getting help from a higher source. These channeling crystals can be used anytime a person is seeking answers or help from outside themselves. It is important to listen very carefully when using these crystals and realize that answers can come from many different sources.

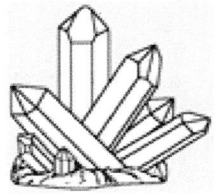
Quartz Clusters

Among other crystals there are quartz clusters which are very healing for all chakras, they bring light into the aura bodies, promote spiritual expansion, awareness, clear negativity on all levels, aid emotional stability, speed up healing, and bring goodness on every level.

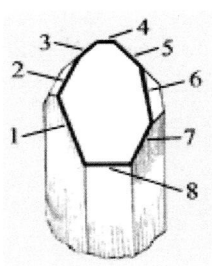
Grounding Crystals

Other special crystals include grounding crystals which have eight edges surrounding the largest sloping face of the crystal. These are rare and are not always easily available. Grounding crystals bring in the ability to deal with practical matters in a realistic way, as they connect people with the earth and keep a person's energies from being scattered. When using grounding crystals, they help people to think clearly and express themselves in a clear way. If these crystals are used during meditation they help a person to form a strong connection with higher knowledge, and keep the person grounded so that the person can apply that information in practical terms. While using a grounding crystal to work through a personal problem, a person should remember that it will require them to look at the truth of the situation and will compel the person to deal with that truth.

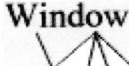
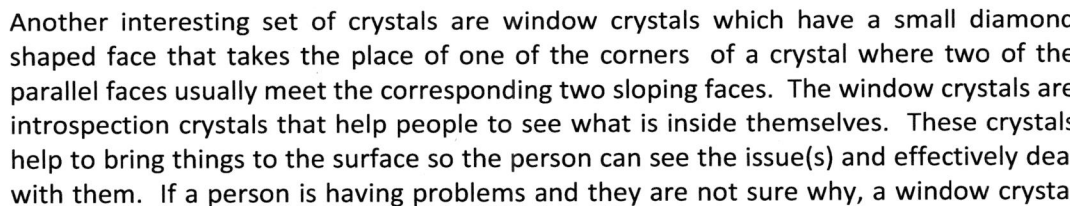
Window Crystals

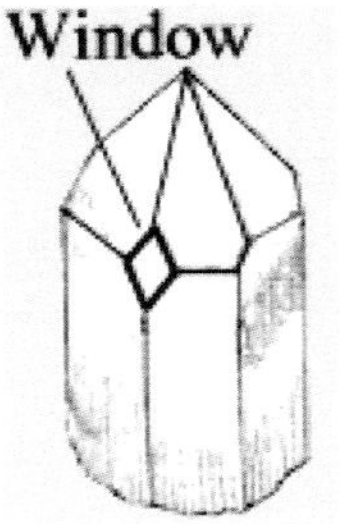

Another interesting set of crystals are window crystals which have a small diamond shaped face that takes the place of one of the corners of a crystal where two of the parallel faces usually meet the corresponding two sloping faces. The window crystals are introspection crystals that help people to see what is inside themselves. These crystals help to bring things to the surface so the person can see the issue(s) and effectively deal with them. If a person is having problems and they are not sure why, a window crystal can be good for figuring out what is going on. Crystal healers will use window crystals for working within themselves to deal with problems and changes that must be made in their lives. Window crystals are used in meditation to help people solve problems that are troubling their Inner Being.

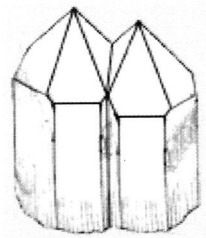
Twin Crystals

Other important crystals include twin crystals which have two terminations (points) at the same end that have developed from a single base. They are called twin crystals because they come from two crystals that are simply attached to each other by the fact that both parts of a twin crystal are exactly parallel to each other and have no boundary between them in at least a small region of the crystal. Twin crystals are nice to work with when dealing with relationship situations. The twin crystals can help people to gain insight into the underlying problems in a relationship, and help work through them. These crystals can generate very positive energy towards improving a relationship, and a twin with a rainbow in it can be very effectively used to project healing energy into a relationship or to keep a good relationship strong. If someone is having a problem with any type of relationship they can sit quietly with the twin crystal and ask for help, the answers to the questions can come from many directions.

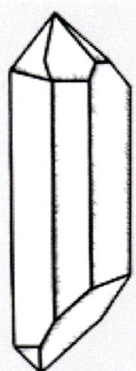
Double Terminated Crystals

Here is another set of interesting crystals which are the double terminated crystals that have points on both ends, allowing energy to flow readily in both directions. The double terminated crystals strengthen energy flow, and are especially useful when a person needs to share or exchange energy between themselves and another person. These crystals are useful when a person is working to help other people, for example in massage or counseling, where energy needs to flow in both directions. In these types of situations, energy flows towards the person when they tune in to another person to find out what that person needs, and energy flows from the healer themselves when they give the person the needed healing energy. The double terminated crystals help to teach the concept of sharing through energy exchange.

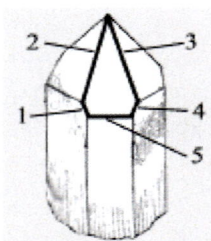
Isis Crystals

Isis crystals have five edges surrounding the largest sloping face of the crystal. The Isis crystals strongly amplify feminine energy, and can help a person to get in touch with the "female" or unselfish side of themselves, no matter whether the person is a man or a woman. If working with Isis crystals they are useful in balancing a person's male-female energy if the female energy has been suppressed, or if the person needs a greater balance of female energy for any reason. The Isis crystals put a person in touch with the power of the Goddess. For men, the Isis crystals will help them to become more in tune with their feminine side and to become more aware of the aspects of women that they may find troubling. As for women, the Isis crystals will help them to regain some of the power and energy that society has taken away from them. These Isis crystals teach that feminine energy is not weak and that anyone doing healing work with another person needs the Isis energy to be effective. The Isis crystals should be carried or held when dealing with issues that are emotional and difficult.

Do some research on the types of crystals you are going to buy so you know what they look like, and about their healing and metaphysical properties for your specific needs. Crystal stores and lapidary suppliers sell a lot of crystals so it is important to understand what to buy. Figure out your price budget in what you can spend on crystals, often times crystals can be expensive so it is good to know some alternatives to purchase instead if what you are looking for is too expensive or not available.

In the beginning when selecting crystals it is recommended to choose crystals like clear quartz for any type of energy healing or goal setting work since clear quartz is an amplifier crystal and will enhance vibrational energies for whatever purpose it is used for. Clear quartz is also great for clearing away unwanted energy. Other crystals that are commonly used for healing may include rose quartz for heart, love healing and energy purification, amethyst for relieving stress and balancing mood swings, carnelian for boosting energy levels, and citrine for grounding and bringing in stability. As well smoky quartz is good because it helps to relieve depression and it is a grounding crystal used for balancing the aura of the human body.

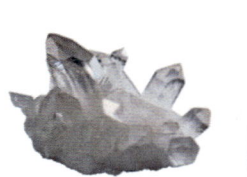 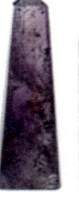 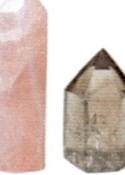 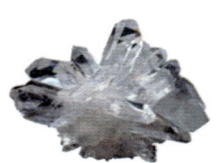

How to Cleanse Crystals?

Although crystals contain their own unique energy vibration, they do absorb the energies of people that handle them and it is a good idea to cleanse the crystals after you acquire them and before you work with them.

Crystal's record and store information so they should also be cleansed after healing sessions. The crystals can pick up energies from other individuals and those energies should not be passed on to other people during healings. If you are using crystals just for yourself then you can cleanse them periodically when needed. On occasions if you have used a crystal for something like healing an emotional hurt it is recommended to cleanse the crystal afterwards so you do not take on the same emotion next time you use that crystal.

There are several methods of how to cleanse crystals. Here are some of these methods:

Thought Energy & Water:

Your crystals can be cleansed by using positive healing light energy which comes from your own mind affirmations or from healing books. Hold the crystal in your hand and visualize cleansing the crystal of all negative energy. You can use an affirmation like "I cleanse and purify this crystal from any unwanted or negative energies. This crystal is now cleansed and purified for the highest good. Amen or Namaste". While visualizing this affirmation you can also put the crystal under running cold water to remove any physical dirt that might be on the crystal(s).

Some crystals that are made of soft minerals should not be washed in water or salt water as well as soap, and detergent because these methods can corrode and break down the composition of the crystals. A few examples of these crystals are pyrite, selenite, amber, turquoise, imperial topaz, red coral, moonstone, opal, all calcites including blue calcite, green calcite, orange calcite, angelite, azurite, kyanite and kunzite or any raw or rough stone.

Sound & Vibration:

Healers can use sound like playing a singing bowl, bells, tingshas, rattle, handpan (metal drum), or drum over or around your crystals to cleanse them with positive melodic vibrational energy. The crystals can be placed on a cloth in the base of a metal singing bowl and then strike the bowl until the sound reaches all its tones for the cleansing process.

Smudging:

Smudge sticks can be used to cleanse crystals. Here are some examples: Cedar, sage, sweet grass, lavender, juniper, pine, Palo Santo.

If using the smudge sticks pass the crystal through the smoke or if you have a large amount of crystals to cleanse then pass the smudge stick over a group of crystals a few times. As you do this "think" away any of the negativity which the crystal may hold. Smudge fans made from feathers are also useful when doing the smudging process to waft the smoke around the crystals. Native Americans use soap stone or red clay bowls that have dried sand in them and on top there is sage placed so when it is lit it creates the smoke to smudge the crystals.

Essential Oils:

Essential oils can act as a cleanser for crystals. The most economical method of using oils is to place crystals in a container, fill it with filtered water and put a drop or two of essential oil into the water. Another method is passing the crystals through vapor made in a burner or vaporizer in which the essential oils are heated.

The following oils can be used:

Lemon: This has a purifying effect and, on a practical level, cuts grease.

Juniper: Like juniper in a smudge stick, juniper oil has the ability to help release any negative vibrations.

Lavender: If you have been doing any kind of intense emotional work with your crystals, lavender oil has a calming and balancing effect. Put some on yourself, too.

Some soft mineral crystals like calcites and selenite cannot be cleansed with essential oils as the oils will seep into the crystal pores and will eventually annul the energies and healing properties of the crystals. It is recommended to refer to a crystal guide book or the internet to see which soft mineral crystals cannot be cleansed with essential oils.

It is a good idea to cleanse tumbled stones with essential oils as these crystals are polished and smooth so they will not corrode or dissolve easily.

Crystals:

Some crystals have the ability to cleanse others. For instance, a carnelian kept in a bag of tumbled crystals will cleanse them and you will never have to cleanse them again. A small crystal, placed on a clear quartz cluster, smoky quartz cluster or amethyst cluster and left overnight will also be cleansed. These cleanser crystals themselves will need cleaning afterwards. The amethyst is said to transform the lower energies of the earth and the universe into the higher frequencies of both the spiritual and the ethereal worlds, therefore cleansing whatever is placed on it. Through research done by crystal healers it has been proven that by using clear quartz, amethyst, and smoky quartz clusters during cleansings that these clusters will assist the stones being cleansed on them in building up their healing energies.

Sunlight/Moonlight:

The rays of the sun and moon are energetically very cleansing, as well as energizing. Placing your crystals outside where they can soak up the sunlight or moonlight for a day or night, or even up to a week is very beneficial.

Sunlight – It is recommended to first rinse the crystals under running water then place them outside in the sun. Research has shown that a good time to cleanse crystals is during a solar eclipse as the vibration from a solar eclipse will charge the crystals with new energy and power.

Moonlight – It is recommended to first rinse the crystals under running water and place them in direct moonlight. As research has shown, it is best to do this method during the Full Moon as it amplifies the healing properties of crystals. Leave the crystals out during the evening to be bathed by the energy of the moon.

Do not put your crystals in the sun too often because the colors of some stones may fade in the sun. A few of the stones that will fade in the sun are amethyst, rose quartz, celestite, opal, and turquoise. If you really want to cleanse the crystals by sunlight, you may choose to place them on a window sill where there is no extreme sunlight but still sufficient sun rays to cleanse them. A good tip to follow is if you are unsure of which crystals to put under the rays of the sun then use the moonlight cleansing method instead.

Reiki Method:

Those of you who practice Reiki healing will know that you can use Reiki energy on almost anything. Reiki energy is not only for humans and animals like pets. Healers can use Reiki energy to purify their food, drinks, plants and also crystals. If you are Reiki Level I you can simply hold a crystal in your hand and Reiki it with universal light energy. Or if you are Reiki Level II you can also draw in the air with your fingers or see in your mind two important symbols that can help to cleanse energy. These images are the mental/emotional symbol of Sei He Ki or distance healing symbol of Hon Sha Ze Sho Nen. Either of these symbols can be drawn or seen in the mind over your crystals in order to give them an advanced form of energy cleansing.

Here is what these symbols look like: **Sei He Ki** 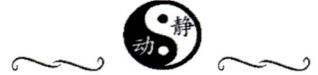   **Hon Sha Ze Sho Nen**

Purpose Made Cleansers:

Purpose Made Cleansers that are made from flower charging essences like Petaltone, Soul Star, White Spring, or Golden Light can be used to cleanse crystals.

Homemade cedar spray with pine or fir can also be used to cleanse crystals, just make sure no acidic essential oils are used in this type of spray. Use a spraying bottle to put the spray in it and mist the crystals from afar lightly with the spray mist. There is no need to use a lot of the spray, a little goes a long way.

When using flower essences you can either place a few drops in a bowl of water and soak or wash your crystals in it or spray the air and pass your crystals through the mist using a solution of water plus 7 drops of the essence in a small spray bottle.

Some soft/soluble crystals like calcites, selenite, or malachite should not be cleansed with Purpose Made Cleansers as this could dissolve these types of crystals. It is recommended to refer to a crystal guide book or the internet to see which soft mineral crystals cannot be cleansed with flower essences.

It is a good idea to cleanse tumbled stones with flower essences as these crystals are polished and smooth so they will not corrode or dissolve easily.

Handling Crystals:

As per proper crystal etiquette it is recommended that if visiting other people's home who have crystals it is a good idea to always ask them permission first if you are allowed to touch or handle their crystals. Sometimes an individual's crystal(s) are reserved for their own personal use. If their crystals are touched or handled by someone else without permission, this could affect the energies a person has programmed into the crystal(s), and could interfere with their connection with the crystal(s) to do healing and manifestation work.

How to Activate and Program Your Crystals?

Crystals can be dedicated and programmed to the purpose for which you use them. Dedicate and program new crystals once you have cleansed them.

When preparing to program your crystal(s) it is important to first make a spiritual connection with your crystal in order to activate it, and to awaken its consciousness. Crystals are historically said to be made out of living matter, since crystals are grown in the earth, they are sentient and have their own living vibration for healing as well as their metaphysical properties.

It is important to be able to visualize the pathways of living energy flowing into your crystal(s), then with your mind's intention focus on the activation of the crystal(s), you may call in your spirit guides, animal totems, angels, and any other light beings to help activate your crystal(s).

Places on earth like vortices, power points like Stonehenge, sacred geometry like pyramids, medicine wheels, sacred locations like Mount Shasta, Sedona Arizona, and special events such as lunar or solar eclipses, or spiritual gatherings like Shaman or Wiccan ceremonies, will help to activate new levels of healing light in your crystal's energy matrix.

When you are getting ready to program a crystal, it is important to dedicate its energies to the highest good of all. While holding the crystal in your hands you can visualize healing white, blue, or golden light surrounding it, and then create your intention for the crystal. It is important to be specific about the purpose in how you want to use the crystal because focused intention is part of the process. Be fully present physically and aware in your mind in the time frame when setting up your purpose/intention for any type of manifestation work. The universe listens to your intention and the message is sent out on the higher planes of existence, and then gets physically manifested on earth.

When you have created your purpose or intention, attune yourself to the crystal; make sure that the crystal you will be working with is exactly the right one for your purpose. The crystal(s) may feel heavy in energy or may seem like it does not have any living energy at all if it is not the right one to use for your purpose/intention.

As you become completely in tune with your crystal(s), you may say out loud or in your mind something like "I program or activate this crystal for/to...[state your purpose]", "I dedicate this crystal to the highest good", "May it be used in light and in love", then you may wear the crystal, position it on your body as appropriate, place it on a crystal grid, put it somewhere in your home where you will see it frequently or keep it in your pocket to manifest the purpose/intention you programmed it with. You can also add a crystal(s) to your water bottle, creating a crystal elixir in order to balance out your energies for positive thinking and behavior.

It is very important to have positive thinking, to be emotionally grounded when programming/activating your crystals. Your mind needs to be clear of any negative thoughts, energies, or distractions that may interfere with creating your purpose/intention for programming your crystals. Before doing any type of crystal programming/activation it is recommended to first ground yourself through meditation or any types of cleansing of your auric fields like smudging yourself and your home with sage, sweet grass, Palo Santo, etc., to create a safe, calm and peaceful environment for programming/activating your crystals.

Meditating with Crystals?

The act of meditation allows a person to attain higher states of consciousness and brings about a greater sense of awareness that enables to see solutions, answers, and insights for everyday life occurrences. During meditation a stone or crystal may be held in the hands or worn when meditating. When wearing or holding crystals their healing and metaphysical properties are being absorbed by the person who is meditating, this helps to create a state of calmness and relaxation both emotionally and physically. A crystal can be held or placed at the heart chakra for emotional balance or third eye chakra for mental clarity during meditation. Crystals can also be programmed to help maintain a deeper level of meditation and sometimes a person may want to create a specific intention and have an outcome during the meditation to accomplish some type of goal. Any type of crystal can be chosen for meditation but quartz crystals are most helpful as they give the person the added advantage of being able to program them more easily than some other stones.

The meditation can last anywhere from ten minutes to an hour depending on how deeply the person goes into the meditative state. It takes time and practice to learn how to meditate and meditating each day for about fifteen minutes will help to center/balance the mind and body in order to have a productive day ahead with happiness and success.

Directions for an Easy Relaxation Meditation:

- Sit on a comfortable chair in a fairly upright position, or on a pillow on the floor, relax your muscles.
- Close your eyes and take a nice slow deep breath in... and as you let it out, allow yourself to completely and fully relax.
- Take another slow deep breath in, and as you let it out feel your body relaxing even more.
- Take a third slow deep breath in, and as you let it out... this time move your awareness to your toes. Tense your toes and your legs, then let go of the tension and relax them fully. As the tension drains away you will feel even more relaxed.

Next place your attention on the area just above your head... and imagine **a ball of golden light** hovering there. Move your attention to that golden light, and allow it to move slowly down into your body. As you take it down through your body... allow the tension to ease from each place that the golden light touches.

- Bring it down through your crown to your third eye... relaxing both your crown and the rest of your head. Move the light down to your throat... and just let any tension there drain away.
- As you bring it to your heart area, allow it to expand out... filling your heart with the loving vibration of Spirit. Fully relax as you allow the golden light to vibrate within you, and feel its loving energy clearing any emotional hurt or pain you may be feeling within your heart.
- Let the light move down through your stomach, filling your solar plexus and sacral areas with this peaceful light.
- Finally take it down to the base of your spine... then down through the base to the earth chakra where you will ground this energy with Mother Gaia.
- Allow this energy to fully ground you to the earth and allow yourself to fully connect to the earth and allow yourself to fully make contact with Mother Gaia and her energy.

Now imagine that this **ball of golden light** is expanding outwards from your body, forming a bubble of light around your entire body. Visualize the golden light flowing out into your entire aura. Allow it to expand out to all the layers of your auric field, energizing you on all levels and totally protecting you.

- Continue to remain with the Golden light filling you for as long as you wish. Allow yourself to simply sit in this lovely relaxed state and let your thoughts float, knowing that this powerful golden light is permeating your complete body, clearing any disharmony within you, and stimulating healing on all levels of your being.

When you are ready just say **'Thank You' to Spirit**, and release the light... and as you do, allow any excess energy to move down to Mother Gaia.

Doing a Crystal Meditation:

- Sit on a comfortable chair in a fairly upright position, or on a pillow on the floor, relax your muscles. Begin by taking a few slow deep breaths in and out. You feel calm and grounded.
- Take a crystal(s) of your choosing into your hands. Put your hands in your lap, focus on the center of the crystal, look within the crystal and imagine yourself stepping inside it. You can close your eyes or leave them open while focusing on the crystal.
- Allow your mind to be clear of any thoughts or feelings.
- Take slow deep breaths in and out, keeping your muscles relaxed.
- Become attuned with the vibrational energies of the crystal. Allow yourself to merge with the crystal and let its healing energies balance your mind and body, become one with this energy.
- Keeping your mind focused on the crystal you may set an affirmation with an intention in creating a program for the crystal during the meditation. The affirmation should use words in the present tense to empower the programming. Here are some examples of affirmations:
    - I feel peaceful and relaxed.
    - I allow myself to be relaxed during meditation.
    - I focus my thoughts in a peaceful and harmonious way.
    - I fill my mind with beautiful thoughts that make me feel happy.

- ♦ My relationships with others are peaceful and productive.
- ♦ I choose for my day to be productive today.
- If you wish you can allow the programming that you have empowered into the crystal to synchronize with your mind and body's energy fields.
- If the programming was for peace and harmony, feel the peace drift through your body… and allow it to take away any tension or stress that may be in any part of your body.
- Take slow deep breaths in and out, let the healing crystal energies take away anything that is not needed, continuing to be aware of any changes anywhere in your body, taking note of them, then letting them go.
- If you would like you may ask the crystal questions about yourself, your life, any issues going on, and about others that are close to you. You can communicate with the crystal and may receive answers from the crystal to help with whatever is going on in your life.
- Spend as much time with the crystal as you need to ask questions, you may also receive images from the crystal and impressions when communicating with it. Take in the information the crystal is sharing with you, and ponder the messages.
- Stay with the energy of the crystal and the empowered programming as long as needed, feeling relaxed and safe, flow with what is happening in the responses of your body.
- Experience the feelings created within you by the crystal, process those feelings, become at peace with your inner self.
- Follow the crystal's energy through all of your body allowing this energy to heal your mind and physical self until you are ready to finish.
- When you are ready give thanks at the end of the meditation to the crystal for its help, and to the Great Divine Spirit for the results you have experienced.

If choosing to meditate with crystals it is important to have a quiet area/space where the person can meditate in peace and silence without interruptions by others. This is integral in order to achieve a state of total relaxation or a dreamlike sensation. It is nice to meditate in an area that is clean and free of clutter, has some type of altar with personal items that mean something to the person meditating like incense candles, flowers, figurines, shells, water feature, pictures, etc. Having these items will bring in positive energy into the meditation space and create a sense of peace, harmony, and joy in the environment. Incorporating soothing meditation music can help with the relaxation process and the facilitation of communicating better with the crystals. Some healers have a whole meditation room devoted to crystals, and this is called a crystal room. A crystal room may create the atmosphere of being in a spa like environment where the healer achieves the highest state of wellbeing.

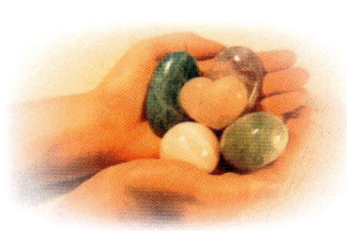 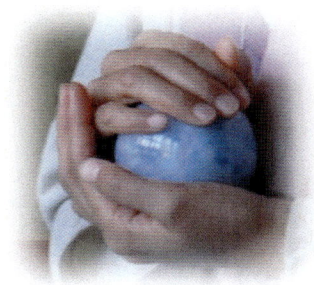 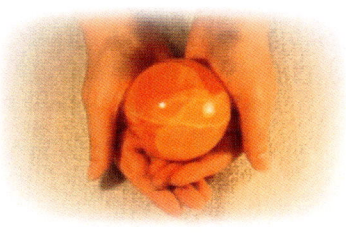

Here are some examples of meditation altars:

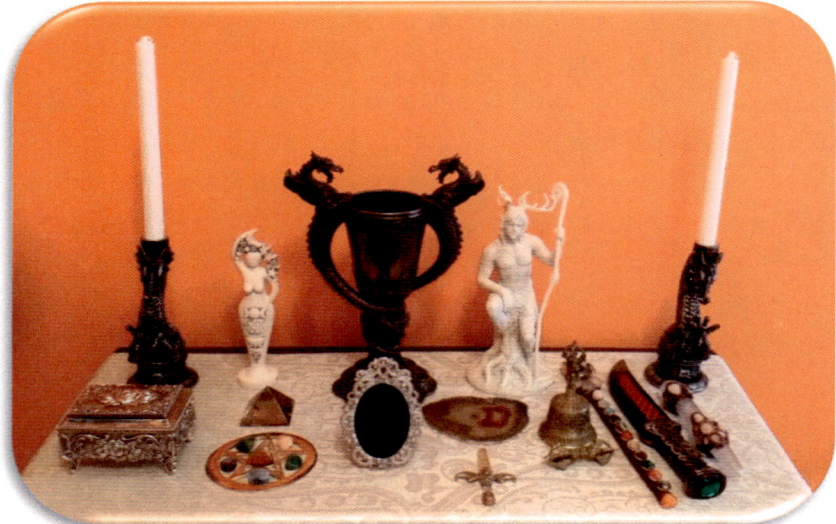

Wiccan Altar honoring the god and the goddess and the elemental forces of the universe. This altar brings in wisdom, ancient knowledge from the universe, and spiritual growth. The altar has an Athame for bringing in energy, Bell for sound cleansing, Black Mirror for scrying, Wands for clearing energies, Crystals for protection, Chalice for ritual work, etc. These are tools that Wiccan's use in their ceremonies and rituals to do magic.

Shamanic Altar honoring the earth, nature, and life force energies sustaining the universe. The way of the shaman offers peace, tranquility, and a balance with life on earth.

This altar brings honor to animals like the eagle, pelican, owl, and butterfly. There are feathers to acknowledge the element of air and the winged beings, sage to honor the element of fire, abalone shell to respect the element of water. The shaman's stone is brown and the jade stones are green representing the element of earth as the cradle of life and civilization. There is a cedar smudge fan for cleansing negative energies from the body and the environment, the fan can either be used to cleanse with water or smoke coming from sage when lit in a soap stone bowl filled with sand.

All these items represent the beauty of living matter and a sense of finding the true self, the inner and outer being becoming one. This altar brings stability and good health to the physical and the emotional sides of a person.

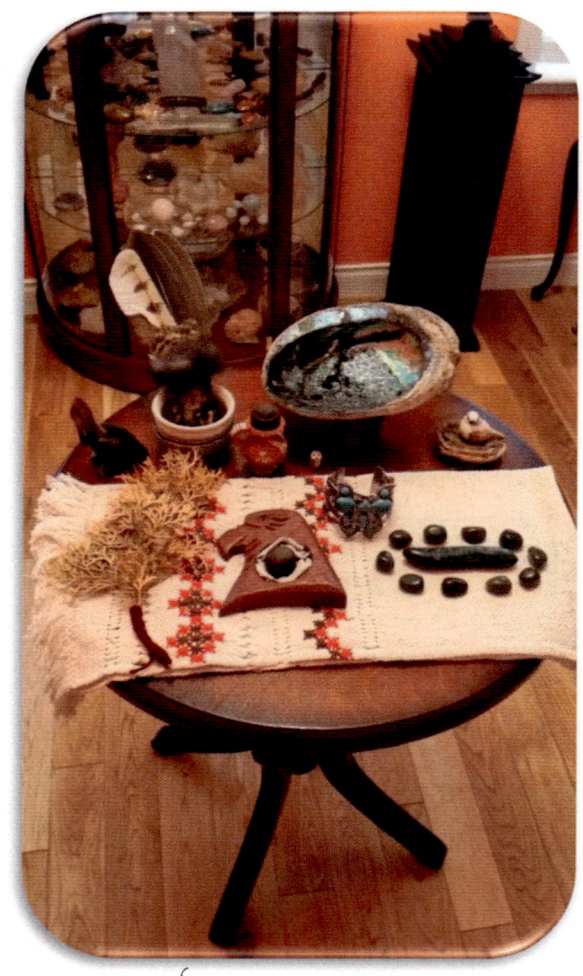

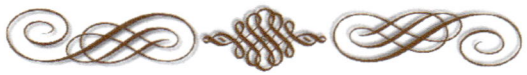

Hand Made Healing Tools & Healing Spaces

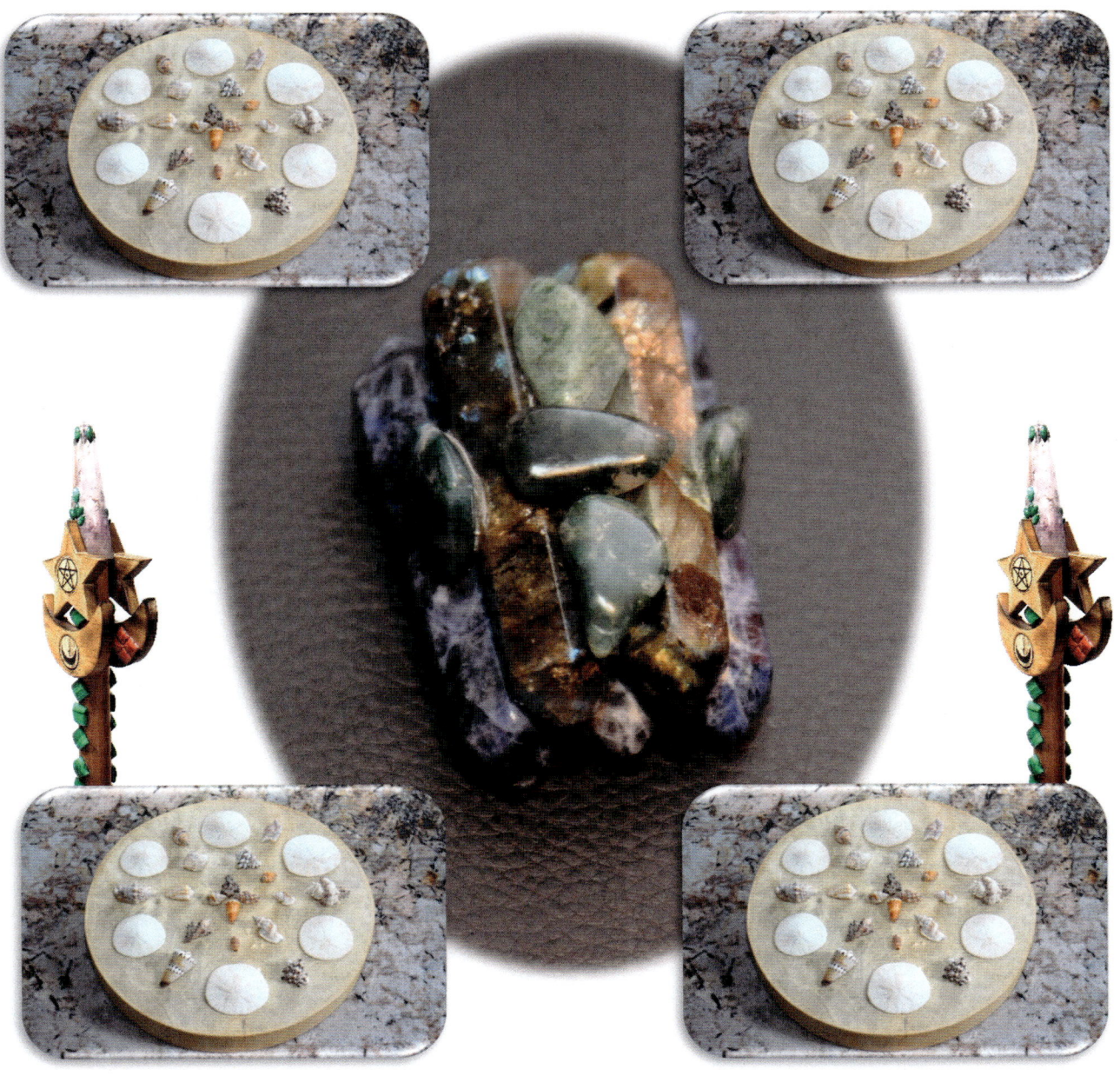

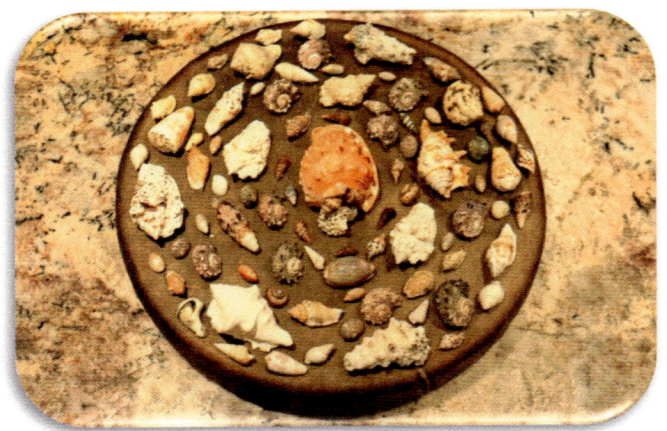
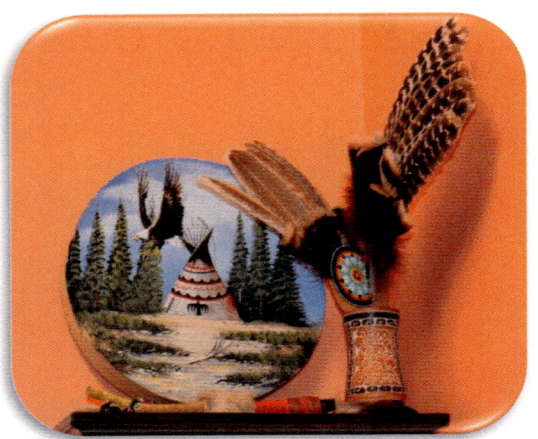
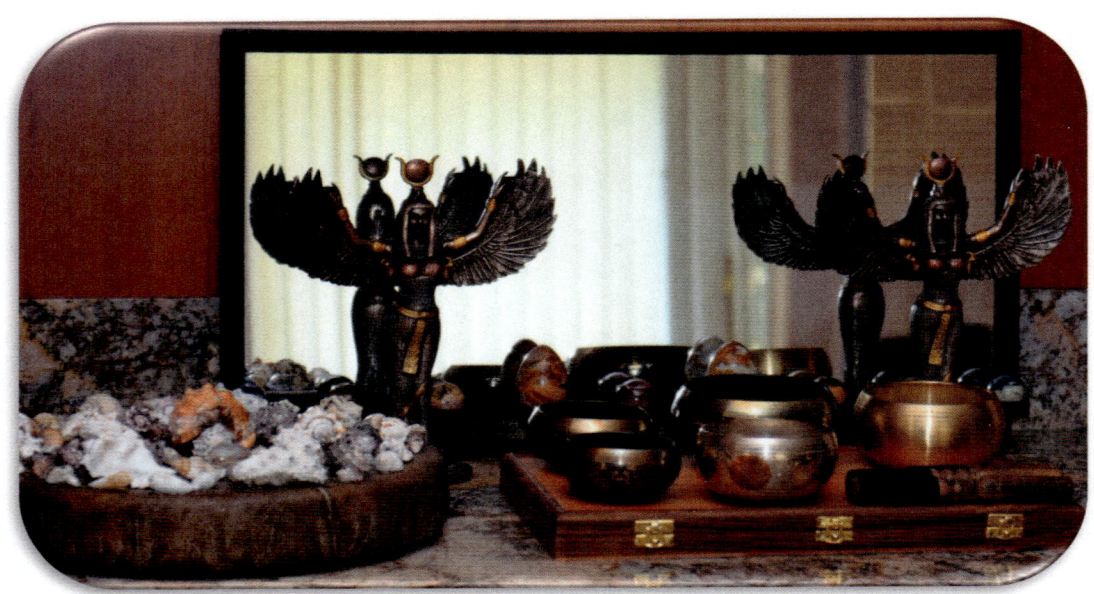

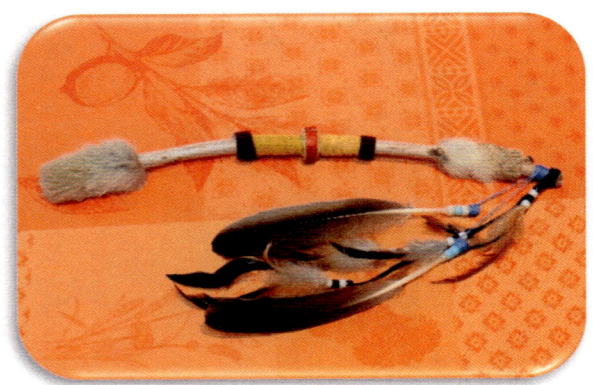

Shaman Talking Stick

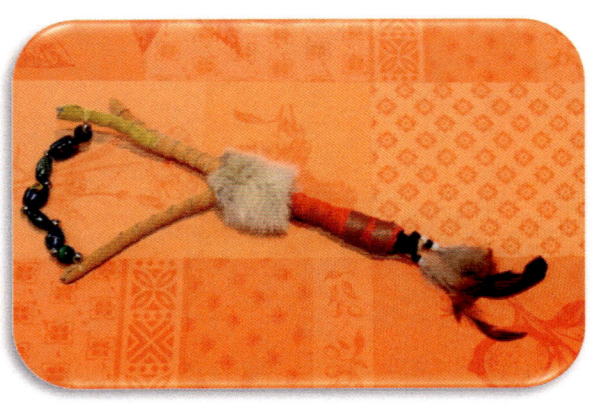

Shaman Rattle